Handstand Mastery:

A Beginner's Guide to learn how to easily do a Handstand

By Steve Plitt

Table of Contents

Copyright

responsibility of the recipient reader.

Under no circumstances will any legal responsibility or blame be held against the publisher for any reparation, damages, or monetary loss due to the information herein, either directly or indirectly.

Respective authors own all copyrights not held by the publisher.

The information herein is offered for informational purposes solely, and is universal as so. The presentation of the information is without contract or any type of guarantee assurance.

The trademarks that are used are without any consent, and the publication of the trademark is without permission or backing by the trademark owner. All trademarks and brands within this book are for clarifying purposes only and are the owned by the owners themselves, not affiliated with this document.

Introduction

I want to thank and congratulate you for purchasing this book *"Handstand Mastery: A Beginner's Guide to Learn How to Easily Do a Handstand"*.

Some people think that doing a handstand is just so easy, but it actually takes a lot of patience and determination in order to do a proper handstand. Handstands are actually beneficial mainly because they can strengthen your core, open up your shoulders, strengthens the back, butt, and legs, as well—so it's definitely good for you!

With the help of this book, you'll learn tips and tricks on how to do the perfect handstand!

Start reading now and find out how!

Chapter 1: Warm up Your Wrists

The very first thing that you have to keep in mind is that you need to warm up your wrists. This means that you have to do wrist or hand exercises that will strengthen your wrists because you need them in order for you to maintain your balance while doing the handstand. Here are some exercises that you could try:

The Fist

- Wrap your thumb around your finger then make a fist and stay in that position for at least a minute or even just 30 seconds.

- After 30 to 60 seconds, release your fingers then repeat the exercise at least three to four times.

Wrist Curls

- Sit down and make sure that your back is straight.

- Then, position your forearms on your thighs.

- Let your thumbs point upwards then get a weight that's around 5 to 20 pounds.

- Now, lift the weight for around 30 seconds back and forth to develop some of your wrist muscles such as the brachioradlis muscle that will help you maintain your balance while doing a handstand.

Finger Curls

- Sit down and get weights that are around 5 to 20 pounds.

- Hold the weight in your hands then hold up your palm upwards and put down your wrist on your thigh. Make sure that the back of your wrist is close to the thigh.

- Let yourself feel the weight of what you have in your hands and once you do so, let your fingers curl so you could feel more weight. This will help you learn how to carry yourself while doing a handstand.

Stretch Your Fingers

- Put your hand down on a flat surface and straighten the fingers as wide and long as possible.

- Hold the position for at least 30 to 60 seconds then repeat for 3 to 4 times more.

Strengthen Your Grip

- Get a soft ball then squeeze it in your palm.

- Keep squeezing for a couple of seconds then repeat the exercise for at least 15 times more for each hand.

Extend Your Thumbs

- Place your hand down on a flat surface, such as a table.

- Then, bring out a rubber band and wrap it around your hands. Make sure that it touches your finger joints, especially the base.

- Now, work in such a way that you get to move your thumbs away from your fingers. Stretch as much as you can and see how far you can go.

- Hold the position for at least 30 seconds before releasing then repeat for 10 times more on each hand.

Wrist Extension

- In coordination with your elbow, extend your wrist for around 30 seconds,
- Do as much as you can for at least 2 minutes so that your forearms will be extended and would be a lot stronger.

Also, in order for you not to have a hard time in doing these exercises, it would be best if you soak your hands in warm water or use a heating pad at least five minutes before doing the exercises. This will make the exercise more effective, too!

Chapter 2: Warm up Your Shoulders

After warming up your wrists, you should also make it a point to warm up your shoulders, as well, because they're important in making sure that your head stays in coordination with your body and that you won't feel easily tired while you're doing a handstand.

Opening up the shoulders is also very important when it comes to doing a proper handstand and there are a couple of exercises that you can do to prepare your shoulders for the handstand. These exercises are:

Tennis Ball Massage

1. Lie face down on a mat then extend one of your arms to the side. Make sure that it's straight.

2. Then, make sure that your elbow on the opposite side of your body is also on the mat.

This will help you become more in control of the exercise.

3. Roll the tennis ball on the muscles of your shoulders then let it roll all the way to your chest.

4. Roll until your find the sensitive area then put some pressure on it until you notice that the tightness has been released.

Tilt Your Head

1. As slow and as carefully as you can, lower your right ear down to your right shoulder.

2. Then, do the same process to your left ear and your left shoulder.

3. Make sure that you once the ear touches the shoulder, you make it a point to end the exercise because you wouldn't want your neck muscles to be ultra-stressed.

4. Do the exercise at least 4 to 5 times for each side of your body.

The Shrug

1. Inhale. As you do so, make sure that your shoulders touch your ears. Do this for around 3 to 4 times.

2. Then, let your shoulders fall as you exhale.

3. Repeat the exercise for at least 4 to 5 times. Aside from relieving muscle tension while you're doing the handstand, this will also help you breathe better so you won't feel like you're gasping for breath.

Open Your Chest

1. Place your hands on your hips and take a deep breath.

2. Then, exhale then lightly tuck your chin in while doing so.

3. As you tuck your chin in, lightly squeeze together your shoulder blades.

4. Repeat for 3 to 4 times more.

Massage the Shoulder

1. Put your left hand on your right shoulder then angle your head to the left.

2. Use your fingers and run them through the shoulder muscles and squeeze your shoulders gently.

3. Do the same exercise to the other part of your body.

Nod Your Head

1. First, angle your chin in such a way that it's tucked on your chest. Do this slowly for around three counts.

2. Be very careful and make sure that your neck is the only part of your body that's moving so that the back muscles will just be steady.

3. Now, lift your head up before facing down, and gaze back at the ceiling. Again, do it slowly so you won't be stressed out.

4. Repeat the exercise for 4 to 5 times more.

Chapter 3: Strengthen Your Core

Another thing that you have to keep in mind is that you have to strengthen your core. Why? Simply because if your core is weak then you really cannot expect yourself to be able to hold the handstand for long. The core pertains to the midsection of your body, particularly the back and abdominal muscles, as well as the glutes and other lower extremities.

In order to strengthen your core, there are a couple of exercises that you can try and here are some of them:

Crunches

To do Crunches, you should:

1. First, lie down with your back on the floor and let your feet rest on a wall.

Bend your knees and hips until they reach a 90-degree angle. This position will then be able to tighten your muscles.

2. Next, work on your shoulders and on your head and lift them up from the floor. Put your arms across your chest then place them beneath your head and hold the position while you are taking around three to four deep breaths.

3. Repeat as necessary.

Abdominal Press

There are two ways of doing the Abdominal Press and these are:

1. Your right hand should be pushed against the left knee then pull your other knee with your free hand. Then, repeat the exercise using your other leg and hand and repeat for at least three to four times.

2. Or, you can also do the exercise by putting one of your hands alongside your left knee then push your leg inwards once more.

This will then be able to help you create resistance especially when your knee is away from the center of your body. Repeat with your other leg and hand for 2 times more.

Double Abdominal Press

Again, there are two ways of doing so, and it's almost the same as Abdominal Press except for the fact that you'd have to use both of your hands and knees at the same time.

What you can do is:

1. First, place each of your hands on the knees opposite them then push inwards. You have to see your arms crossing above each other to know that you're doing the right thing. Hold the position for at least three heavy breaths and repeat for four more times.

2. Another variation would be to just put your hands on the sides of your knees.

Push your knees inward once more then pull them away from the center so you could create some resistance. Repeat for four times more for 3 deep breaths each.

The Bridge

To do this exercise, you should:

1. Lie down on a yoga mat or on the ground with your back flat and while bending your knees. Make sure that your back stays in a neutral position and make sure that you do not tilt your hips.

2. Now, slowly raise your hips from the ground and hold the position for at least three deep breaths then repeat exercise for 3 more times.

The Side Plank

1. To do the side plank, you have to lie down with your left side touching the ground or the yoga mat.

2. Then, allow yourself to raise your body with the help of your left forearm and make sure that your left elbow is under your left shoulder and just let your right arm stay on the other side of your body.

3. Now, squeeze your abdominal muscles together and stay in that position in the duration of three breaths and help yourself pull your balance together with the use of your left hand.

4. Let yourself raise your hips then point your right hand upwards for 3 breaths.

5. Repeat for 2 to 3 times more.

Mister Superman

1. Put a small pillow or a rolled towel on the yoga mat for you to place your hips on to give your back some support.

2. Then, slowly tighten your abdominal muscles and pull your arm upwards so it will point towards the ceiling.

3. As for your other arm, just make sure that it stays down and that you take 3 deep breaths while doing so.

4. Then, finally, allow your left leg to be raised off the floor and just hold your other leg down for 3 deep breaths.

5. Repeat for 2 to 3 times more.

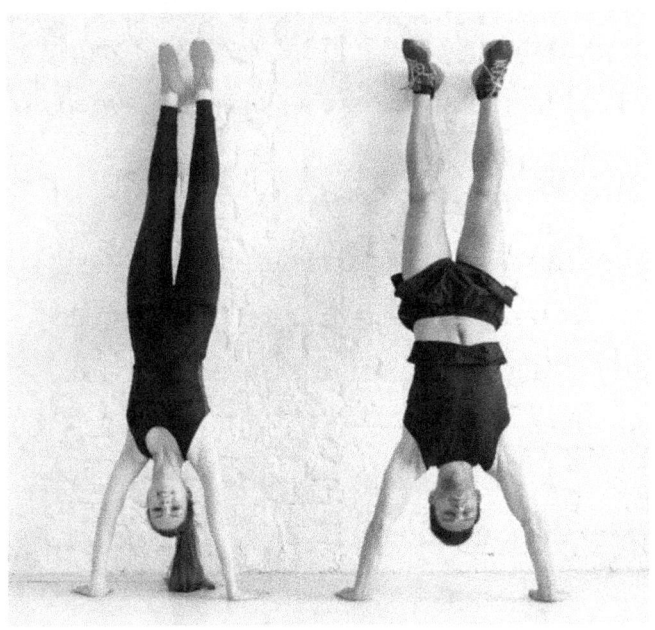

Chapter 4: Position Your Body Properly

Now comes what a lot of people refer to as the tricky part. You have to learn how to position your body in such a way that it would help you maintain composure as you're doing the handstand.

There are a couple of positions that you have to put into practice so that you can properly do the handstand. Here's what you have to do.

The Hollow Body

The Hollow Body is considered as the basic handstand position because it helps you do the "straight handstand" stance. To do this, you have to:

1. Lie down on a yoga mat with your back flat on the ground.

2. Then, let your lower back touch the ground so you can angle your belly button downwards.

3. Tighten your abs and your butt then point your arms straight upward and keep your toes pointed.

4. Raise your shoulders and legs off the ground then let your ears stay with your shoulders. At the same time, make sure that your abs and butt are still tight but make sure that they don't touch the ground.

5. Slowly lift your arms higher—just do it however you can and hold the position for a couple of seconds or so. This way, your body will be "hollow" and you'll be ready to do the handstand.

The Hands

As mentioned earlier, your hands are key to a successful handstand and that's why you were asked to warm them up.

After the warm-up, it's time for you to position your hands the way they're meant to be when it comes to a handstand.

Here's how:

1. First, make sure that you stretch out your hands and that they're at least apart from each other by a shoulder-width length.
2. Splay your fingers open wide. Don't keep them close together because this would not help you maintain your balance and you have to keep them open wide so you'd get a whole lot of support from them.
3. Then, firmly press your palms onto the floor as a starting position.

The Elbows

Next up are the elbows. You also have to make sure that you follow each procedure carefully as this is crucial for the handstand.

Here's what you have to do:

1. First, screw your shoulders inward so that you'll see that your elbow pit is inching forward.
2. Keep your elbows straight because if you bend them just a tiny bit, you'll be tired because it means that your muscles will do a lot of work—and that's not what you want to happen.

The Shoulders

Next up are your shoulders. The main idea is for them to be hugging your ears and that they have to be really elevated.

Here's how you can help yourself get in this position:

1. At first, you may need to stand on a tubing and then try to squeeze your shoulders to your head and make sure that you push your arms overhead.

2. As you do this, make sure that you angle your elbows the way you were taught earlier. It's essential that you work on the shoulders and elbows at the same time.

The Lower Body

While some people think that the lower body has nothing to do with a handstand, experts agree that it is a big deal and that it plays a big role— so you have to know how to position it well. Here's what you have to do:

1. Make sure that you bring your feet together and that they are in a pointed position.

2. As for your legs, you have to squeeze them together, as well. Do it as tight as you can because the tighter your lower body is, the better, as you'd be able to better hold your balance. The key is to remember to "squeeze" and not flail or let your lower body open wide. This would help you be more flexible and make the handstand stable.

The Head

As for the head, it's important to keep things neutral. This means that it should just be hanging and that you don't let it touch the ground—or else all the blood will go to your head and you definitely won't feel good.

And, breathe

And of course, in doing a handstand, it's so important that you breathe properly. Handstand masters agree that its best that you recite your favorite quotes or even sing while you're doing the handstand so that you won't feel so pressured and you'd be able to breathe properly. Here are some breathing exercises that you could try:

1. Use your nose to take deep breaths in so that the diaphragm will be inflated and your chest won't have to work so much. Six to ten deep breaths will already do you a lot of good.

2. Before doing the handstand, you can also make it a point to do a meditative breathing exercise each day. You can do so by holding your thumb over your nostril then inhale through your other nostril. Do this for 10 seconds before moving on to the other nostril. Repeat for around 3 to 4 times.

3. You can also try inhaling slowly then release your breath in a fast manner. This will help you deal with being in an unusual position, such as a handstand, and it will also perk you up so you'd feel energized!

4. Just visualize. Think of your happy place, think of things that calm you down and make you feel better and surely, you'll be able to breathe. Remember that there is no room for anxious thoughts right now.

Now that you know how to position your body, it's high time for you to learn how to do the various kinds of handstands. Flip to the next chapter and find out how!

Chapter 5: Basic Types of Handstands

As mentioned earlier, there isn't just one kind of handstand—there are actually a lot and that's great because at least, you can find something that you feel is most suitable for you! Here they are.

The Straight Handstand

Others call this "Hollow Body" or "Facing the Wall", but basically, it's the first type of handstand that you have to learn as it's most suited for beginners. To do this, you have to:

1. First, put your hands on a yoga mat or on the ground then allow your feet to rest on the wall.

2. Make sure that your legs and feet are squeezed together and they are pointing upwards.

3. Allow your hands to get close to the wall, as well then let your feet go on a 90

degree angle while the balls of your feet are close to the wall.

4. Look at the wall while your chin is tucked in then remember the hollow body exercise that you made earlier and tighten your butt and abs.

5. Point your arms down while keeping your toes pointed upwards.

6. Do this for at least 30 seconds and repeat for around 8 times.

Twisted Straight

This is almost like the Straight Handstand, except for the fact that now, you have to face away from the wall.

To do this, you should:

1. Put your hands on a yoga mat or on the ground then allow your feet to rest on the wall.

2. Make sure that your legs and feet are squeezed together and they are pointing upwards.

3. Face away from the wall. You can do so by kicking a leg up or jump and arch your body to the wall.

4. Then, let your lower back touch the ground a bit so you can angle your belly button downwards.

5. Tighten your abs and your butt then point your arms straight down and keep your toes pointed.

6. Raise your shoulders and legs off the ground then let your ears stay with your shoulders. At the same time, make sure that your abs and butt are still tight but make sure that they don't touch the ground.

7. Allow your arms to touch the ground as much as you can and allow your shoulders to be extended.

8. Repeat the process for around 8 times with holding times of at least 30 seconds each.

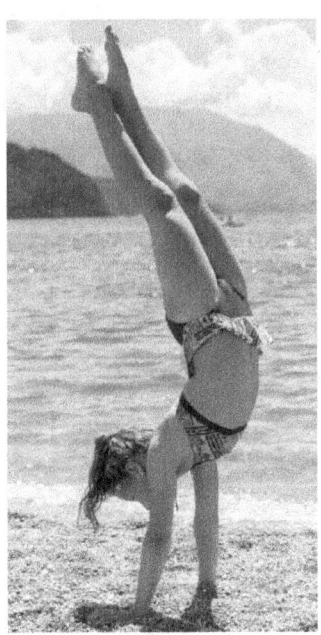

L is the Name

The final basic type of handstand is called the "L". What's great about this is that it strengthens your core more than other types of handstands can. You can do so by:

1. Angle your body in a 90 degree position, or an "L" position as your feet are touching the wall.

2. Make sure that your butt are over your shoulders to make the perfect "L" then tighten your upper body so that it would be able to give you a lot of support.

3. Now, as for your head, you just have to look straight to the wall then let yourself kick one leg up then work to push your body away from the wall, slowly. After doing so, you should see that both of your legs are now on top of you.

To get out of any handstand, it would be safe to do a cartwheel so that you can get out of the position.

Once you have mastered the basic types of handstands, you can move on to more complex ones but you have to remember that you can't try them out right away. These includes one-arm handstands, Mexican handstands, Split handstands, and the like. While they may tempt you to try them right away, you have to realize that you can't do them yet because you need to practice more and you have to make sure that you have mastered the basic handstands first. It might take weeks, months, or even years to progress—so focus on these basic ones first.

Chapter 6: Other Reminders

Now that you know how to warm yourself up before a handstand and how to do a proper handstand, you should also be aware of the other things that you have to know about when it comes to doing a handstand so you can do it well and you won't feel tired easily.

Here are the other things that you have to keep in mind:

1. **Do some Weight Training.** Weight Training is important if you want to make sure that you're able to do your handstands properly simply because weight training exercises can strengthen your core, your arms, and your shoulders. Some of the exercises that you can try include military or overhead presses. Do these at least two to three times a week and surely, you'll have the perfect stance for doing handstands.

2. **Learn how to Traverse.** Another thing that can really help you when it comes to doing proper handstands is the ability to traverse or walk from one side of the wall to the other while you're doing a handstand. To do so, just do a straight handstand position where you are facing the wall and just allow your feet to rest on the wall. Now, after you have done so, use your hands in such a way that you would use your feet for walking then walk as much as you can. If you feel like you can't walk too far on your first attempt, don't worry about it because it's normal. Just do whatever you can so on your next practice, you'd be able to do more and so on.

3. **Do Push-ups.** Push-ups are very helpful especially while you're doing a handstand because they'd help you concentrate better. To do so, while you're doing a handstand, just make sure that your toes don't come close to the floor then just push your hands

towards the ground, like you're doing a regular push-up except from the fact that you're currently standing. Push your arms and fingers down, straighten your back, point your toes, and make sure to shrug your shoulders, too. This way, you get to improve your balance and flexibility. Push-ups will also strengthen your spinal and neck columns and improve the way you carry your body weight not just while you're doing a handstand but also while you're doing things that you normally do.

Now, keep on pushing down the way you would a regular push-up. You can also play around by traversing or going in the L-position to give yourself a bit of a challenge and to make sure that you get to help yourself hold the handstand, whatever kind of handstand it might be.

Also, it would be best not to try headstands because they won't be helpful and they're really not recommended—unless you're trying to show off.

4.   Do some Pull-ups. Pull-ups are beneficial because they can strengthen your back muscles the way no other type of exercise regimen can. For around 5 to 10 minutes each day, allow some time for yourself to do some pull-ups for a month and you will definitely be able to improve your stance. In order to challenge yourself more, it would also be good if you could hold a dumbbell between your legs, or carry a bag filled with books while you're doing the push-ups so the experience will be more intense!

Aside from the fact that you'll be able to do amazing handstands, you'll also be able to do great latches, muscle-ups, and climb-ups, as well, which in turn will help you become efficient when it comes to wall, rock, or mountain climbing, too!

5. Make use of Paralletes. One more way of helping yourself do the perfect handstand is by making use of Paralletes because experts agree that if you can actually hold your balance while using Paralettes then you won't have a hard time doing a perfect handstand— whether or not you're close to the wall.

Paralletes are like mini-tubes or bars that you can make and can hold on to. You can make them by using PVC pipes, end caps, primer, glue, tape measure, fine tooth saw, wire brush, rags, newspaper, and electrical; tape. There are a lot of tutorials that you may find online so check those out. Those Paralletes will come in handy, too, if you want to do more weight training.

6. And, don't forget that practice makes perfect. Some Handstand

Experts have said that there are people who have perfected handstands in a matter of 14 weeks because they made it a point to practice each day. Because realistically speaking, if you don't practice then you really cannot expect that you'll be good at something, can you? Here are some of the things that you have to keep in mind for you to be able to practice well:

a. Each day, give some time for practice. And you have to be consistent about it. It won't actually be hard if you do it each day.

b. Never forget to warm up before practicing. In earlier chapters, you were taught how to warm the important parts of your body up, so make sure that you do just that so your body won't be shocked at how handstands feel.

c. Don't assume that you know everything right away. As mentioned earlier, you have to start with the basics because they will improve your stance and help you understand what to do next.

d. And, work on your own pace. If you're practicing handstands with other people and you feel like they improve faster than you, just focus on the fact that handstands are not about who gets ahead first or who knows what to do right away—it's about trying to improve each day and making sure that you're doing the right thing. And if you practice constantly, then you most certainly will be able to do proper handstands!

Conclusion

Thank you for reading this book.

I hope this book was able to help you understand what a handstand is and how you can do a proper one.

The next step is to make sure that you follow the techniques given in this book and you'll surely perfect the art of doing handstands!

Finally, if you enjoyed this book, please take time to post a review on Amazon. It will be greatly appreciated.

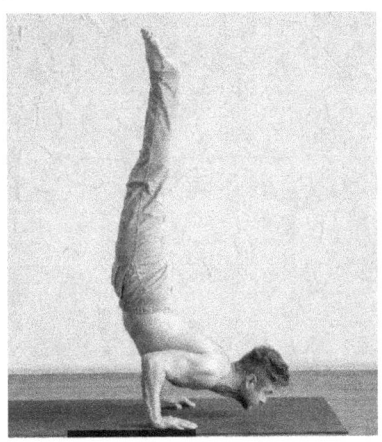

www.ingramcontent.com/pod-product-compliance
Lightning Source LLC
Chambersburg PA
CBHW070507290526
45790CB00003B/1127